What is HIV treatment?

HIV treatment (antiretroviral treatment or Workmanship) includes accepting medication as endorsed by a medical services supplier. HIV treatment diminishes how much HIV in your body and assists you with remaining solid.
There is no solution for HIV, yet you have some control over it with HIV treatment.
The vast majority can fix the infection in six months or less.
HIV treatment doesn't forestall transmission of other physically communicated illnesses.

When would it be a good idea for me to begin HIV treatment?

Begin HIV treatment as quickly as time permits after determination.

- All individuals with HIV ought to take HIV treatment, regardless of how long they've had HIV or how solid they are.

- Converse with your medical care supplier about any ailments or different prescriptions you are taking.

Consider the possibility that I defer HIV treatment.

Assuming you defer treatment, HIV will keep on hurting your resistant framework. Postponing therapy will put you at a higher gamble for sending HIV to your accomplices, becoming ill, and creating Helps.

Are there various kinds of HIV treatment?

There are two kinds of HIV treatment: pills and shots.

- Pills are suggested for individuals who are simply beginning HIV treatment. There are numerous FDA-supported single pill and mix prescriptions accessible.

- Individuals who have had an imperceptible viral burden (or have been virally smothered) for something like three months might think about shots.

What are HIV treatment shots?

HIV treatment shots are long-acting infusions used to treat individuals with HIV. The shots are given by your medical services supplier and require routine office visits. HIV treatment shots are allowed one time per month or when each and every other month, contingent upon your treatment plan.

Might I at any point change my HIV treatment from pills to shots?

Converse with your medical services supplier about changing your HIV therapy plan. Shots might be ideal for you in the event that you are a grown-up with HIV who

- has an imperceptible viral burden (or has accomplished viral concealment),

- has no set of experiences of treatment disappointment, and
- has no known sensitivity to the prescriptions in the shot.

On the off chance that you and your medical services supplier choose to change your HIV therapy from pills to shots, you'll have to visit your supplier routinely to accept your shots. Tell your medical services supplier quickly on the off chance that you've missed or plan to miss an arrangement for your shot.

What are the advantages of accepting my HIV treatment as endorsed?

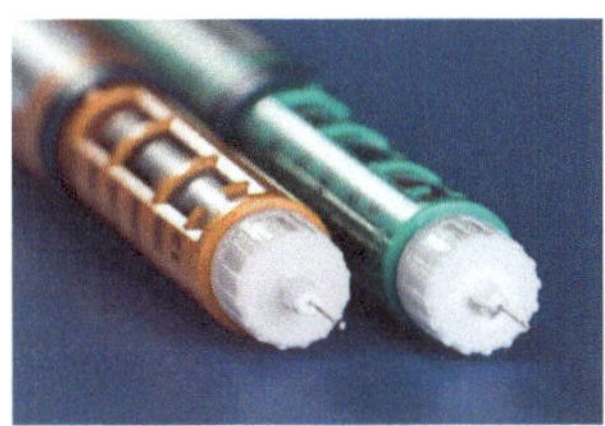

HIV treatment lessens how much HIV in the blood (viral burden).

- Taking your HIV medication as endorsed will assist with keeping your viral burden low.

- HIV treatment can make the viral burden extremely low (popular concealment). Viral concealment implies having under 200 duplicates of HIV for each milliliter of blood.

- HIV treatment can make the viral burden so low that a test can't distinguish it (imperceptible viral burden).

- Assuming your viral burden goes down in the wake of beginning HIV treatment, that implies treatment is working. Keep on accepting your HIV treatment as endorsed.

- In the event that you skirt your HIV treatment, even now, you are allowing HIV the opportunity to quickly duplicate. This could debilitate your invulnerable framework, and you could end up being wiped out.

- Getting and keeping an imperceptible viral burden (or remaining virally stifled) is the most effective way to remain solid and safeguard others.

HIV treatment forestalls transmission to other people.

- In the event that you have an imperceptible viral burden, you won't send HIV through sex. This is otherwise called Imperceptible = Untransmittable.

- Having an imperceptible viral burden probably diminishes the gamble of HIV transmission through sharing needles, needles, or other infusion hardware (for instance, cookers), yet we don't be aware by how much.

- Having an imperceptible viral burden likewise forestalls perinatal transmission. In the event that an individual with HIV takes their HIV medication as recommended all through pregnancy and labor and gives HIV treatment to their child for 4 to about a month and a half after birth, the gamble of transmission can be 1% or less.

- Having an imperceptible viral burden incredibly decreases the gamble of sending HIV through breastfeeding yet doesn't wipe out the gamble. The ongoing proposal in the US is that guardians with HIV shouldn't breastfeed their children.

Taking your HIV medication as recommended forestalls drug opposition.

- Drug obstruction is created when individuals with HIV don't accept their pills as endorsed or miss their shots. The infection can change (transform) and may restrict your choices for effective HIV treatment.

- Assuming you foster medication obstruction, it will restrict your choices for fruitful HIV treatment.

- Drug-safe kinds of HIV can be communicated to other people.

Does HIV treatment cause secondary effects?

HIV treatment can cause aftereffects in certain individuals. Nonetheless, not every person encounters incidental effects. The most widely recognized incidental effects are:

- Queasiness and regurgitating
- Looseness of the bowels
- Trouble resting
- Dry mouth
- Migraine
- Rash
- Wooziness
- Exhaustion
- Transitory agony at the infusion site (for shots)

Converse with your medical services supplier assuming your HIV therapy makes you wiped out. Your medical care supplier might recommend extra prescriptions to assist with dealing with the secondary effects or may change your HIV therapy plan.

How would it be a good idea for me to respond in the event that I'm contemplating having a child?

Inform your medical services supplier as to whether you or your accomplice is pregnant or pondering getting pregnant. They will decide the right sort of HIV treatment to assist with forestalling passing HIV to your child.

Could I at any point take conception prevention while on HIV treatment?

You can utilize a technique for contraception to forestall pregnancy. Nonetheless, some HIV treatment might make chemical based conception prevention less successful. Converse with your medical services supplier about which strategy for anti-conception medication is appropriate for you.

Will HIV treatment impede my chemical treatment?

Most HIV treatment can be utilized securely with orientation confirming or menopausal chemical treatment and testosterone substitution treatment. Notwithstanding, aftereffects might happen. Converse with your medical care supplier about taking HIV therapy and chemical treatment simultaneously. Your medical care supplier will screen any secondary effects and assist with ensuring your HIV therapy and chemical treatment keep focused.

Imagine a scenario in which my HIV treatment isn't working.

- Your medical care supplier might change your sort of HIV therapy.

- A change is entirely to be expected on the grounds that a similar HIV treatment doesn't influence everybody similarly.

Adhering to my HIV treatment plan is hard. How might I manage the difficulties?

Tell your medical services supplier immediately in the event that you're experiencing difficulty adhering to your arrangement. Together you can recognize the reasons you're skipping HIV treatment and choose how to address those reasons.

Converse with your medical care supplier about issues taking your HIV therapy.

- **Issues taking pills. This can make remaining on this sort of HIV treatment testing. Your medical services supplier can offer methods for resolving these issues, including changing to an injectable HIV therapy choice.**

- **Incidental effects. Sickness or looseness of the bowels can make an individual not have any desire to proceed with their HIV therapy. There are medications or other help, as dietary advising, to ensure you're getting significant supplements. This can assist with the most widely recognized incidental effects.**

- **HIV treatment exhaustion.** Certain individuals find that adhering to their HIV treatment plan becomes more earnest after some time. Make it a highlight to converse with your medical services supplier about remaining on your arrangement.

- **A bustling timetable.** Work or travel away from home can make it simple to neglect to take pills or miss a shot. Keeping additional pills at work or in your car might be conceivable. In any case, converse with your medical services supplier first as outrageous temperatures can influence some medication.

Converse with your medical care supplier in the event that you miss portions of your HIV therapy.

- **Missing a portion of pills.** By and large, you can accept your pills when you understand you missed a portion. Then take the following portion at your typically planned time (except if your drug specialist or medical care supplier has told you in any case).

- **Missing a shot.** On the off chance that you missed an arrangement for your shot, converse with your medical care supplier about accepting your next shot.

- **Missing doses.** Converse with your medical care supplier or drug specialist about ways of assisting you with recollecting your HIV therapy. Your medical services supplier might try and choose to change your therapy to meet your requirements and life circumstances.

Find help for psychological well-being or substance use issues.

- **Being debilitated or discouraged.** What you feel intellectually and truly can mean for your capacity to adhere to your HIV treatment plan. Your medical services supplier, social specialist, or caseworker can allude you to an emotional well-being supplier or nearby care group.

- **Substance use (medication or liquor).** On the off chance that substance use is obstructing your capacity to keep yourself solid, it could be an ideal opportunity to track down help.

- Assuming you want assistance finding substance use, jumble treatment or psychological wellness administrations.

Join a care group or ask your loved ones for help. They can assist you with adhering to your treatment plan.

Living with HIV

HIV and Sustenance and Food handling

Central issues

- In individuals with HIV, great nourishment upholds general wellbeing and keeps up with the resistant framework. Great sustenance likewise assists individuals with HIV keep a sound weight and retain HIV drugs.

- Food and water can be defiled with microbes that cause sicknesses (called foodborne ailments or food contamination).

- Since HIV harms the resistant framework, foodborne illnesses are probably going to be more serious and last longer in individuals with HIV than in individuals with a sound safe framework.

- Sanitation is about how to choose, handle, get ready, and store food to forestall foodborne illnesses. Observing sanitation rules lessens the gamble of foodborne diseases.

For what reason is great sustenance significant for individuals living with HIV?

Great sustenance is tied in with finding and keeping a smart dieting style. Great sustenance upholds generally speaking wellbeing and keeps up with the insusceptible framework. It likewise assists individuals with HIV to keep a solid weight and retain HIV medications.

HIV assaults and obliterates the insusceptible framework, which makes it harder for the body to ward off diseases. Individuals with HIV take a mix of HIV meds (called a HIV treatment routine) consistently. The medications keep HIV from annihilating the invulnerable framework. A sound eating routine likewise reinforces the resistant framework and keeps individuals with HIV solid.

What is a sound eating routine for individuals living with HIV?

By and large, the essentials of a solid eating regimen are no different for everybody, incorporating individuals with HIV.

- Eat various food sources from the five nutrition classes: organic products, vegetables, grains, protein food sources, and dairy.

- Eat the perfect proportion of food to keep a sound weight.

- Pick food varieties low in soaked fat, sodium (salt), and added sugars.

HIV and HIV medications can in some cases cause nourishment related issues. For instance, some HIV-related contaminations can make it hard to eat or swallow. Incidental effects from HIV drugs, like loss of hunger, sickness, or looseness of the bowels, can make it hard to adhere to a HIV routine. In the event that you have HIV and are having a sustenance related issue, converse with your medical services supplier.

To keep away from sustenance related issues, individuals with HIV should likewise focus on food handling.

What is food sanitation?

Food and water can be defiled with microorganisms that cause diseases (called foodborne illnesses or food contamination). Sanitation is about how to choose, handle, get ready, and store food to forestall foodborne diseases.

For what reason is food handling significant for individuals living with HIV?

Since HIV harms the safe framework, foodborne diseases are probably going to be more serious and last longer in individuals with HIV than in individuals with a sound resistant framework. Adhering to food handling rules diminishes the gamble of foodborne illnesses.

What steps can individuals with HIV take to forestall foodborne diseases?

Assuming you have HIV, keep these food handling rules to diminish your gamble of foodborne ailments:

Try not to eat or drink the accompanying food sources:

- Crude eggs or food varieties that contain crude eggs, for instance, custom made treat mixture

- Crude or half-cooked poultry, meat, and fish

- Unpasteurized milk or dairy items and natural product juices

Follow the four fundamental stages to food handling: perfect, isolated, cook, and chill.

- **Clean**: Clean up, cooking tools, and ledges frequently while getting ready food varieties.

- **Isolated**: Separate food varieties to keep the spread of any microbes starting with one food then onto the next. For instance, keep crude meat, poultry, fish, and eggs separate from food varieties that are prepared to eat, including organic products, vegetables, and breads.

- **Cook**: Utilize a food thermometer to ensure that food varieties are cooked to safe temperatures.

- **Chill**: Refrigerate or freeze meat, poultry, eggs, fish, or different food sources that are probably going to pamper in no less than 2 hours of cooking or buying.

HIV Test Precision: Which Sort of Test Is Ideal?

After a potential HIV openness, hanging tight for your experimental outcomes can be a nail-gnawing experience. Might it be said that you are prepared to know your HIV status? Is your life going to change?

When you really do come by the outcomes, how might you be certain they're dependable? Discovering that you tried positive, just to find half a month after the fact that you're really negative — or the other way around — could be a horrible encounter.

Obtaining an exact outcome is significant, for your inner harmony, yet with the goal that you can begin on HIV treatment assuming your experimental outcome is positive or do whatever it may take to forestall future HIV procurement on the off chance that your experimental outcome is negative.

How Exact Are HIV Tests?

All HIV tests supported by the U.S. Food and Medication Organization are extremely exact. All things considered, the specific degree of exactness can shift from one test to another relying upon a couple of variables, most prominently:

- HIV test type

- Whether it's a quick test or a lab test

- How as of late you were presented to HIV

- How your body answers another HIV disease (i.e., creates antibodies)

What sorts of tests are accessible, and how would they work?

There are three sorts of HIV tests: neutralizer tests, antigen/counter acting agent tests, and nucleic basic analyses (NAT). Antibodies are created by your insusceptible framework when you're presented to infections like HIV. Antigens are unfamiliar substances that make your resistant framework actuate. Assuming that you have HIV, an antigen called p24 is created even before antibodies create.

HIV tests are normally performed on blood or oral liquid. They may likewise be performed on pee.

A Counter Acting Agent Test

A counter acting agent test searches for antibodies to HIV in your blood or oral liquid.

- Most fast tests and the main HIV individual test supported by the U.S. Food and Medication Organization (FDA) are neutralizer tests.

- **By and large, neutralizer tests that utilize blood from a vein can distinguish HIV sooner than tests finished with blood from a finger stick or with oral liquid.**

Antigen/Counter acting agent Test

An antigen/immunizer test searches for both HIV antibodies and antigens.

- **Antigen/counter acting agent tests are suggested for testing done in labs and are normal in the US. This lab test includes drawing blood from a vein.**

- **There is likewise a fast antigen/immune response test accessible that is finished with blood from a finger stick.**

Nucleic Basic analysis (NAT)

A NAT searches for the genuine infection in the blood.

- **With a NAT, the medical care supplier will draw blood from your vein and send the example to a lab for testing.**

- **This test can figure out whether an individual has HIV or how much infection is available in the blood (HIV viral burden test).**

- **A NAT can recognize HIV sooner than different kinds of tests.**

- **This test ought to be considered for individuals who have had a new openness or a potential openness and have early side effects of HIV and who have tried negative with an immune response or antigen/neutralizer test.**

Converse with your medical care supplier about what kind of HIV test is appropriate for you.

What amount of time will it require to get my HIV test results?

It relies upon the sort of HIV test and where you get tried.

- **HIV individual tests give results in 20 minutes or less.**

- With a fast immune response test, typically finished with blood from a finger stick or with oral liquid, results are prepared quickly or less.

- The quick antigen/neutralizer test, finished with blood from a finger stick, requires 30 minutes or less.

- It might require a few days to accept your test results with a NAT or antigen/immunizer lab test.

Could a HIV at any point test distinguish the infection following openness?

No HIV test can distinguish HIV following contamination. That is a result of the window time frame — the time between HIV openness and when a test can recognize HIV in your body. The window time frame relies upon the sort of HIV test. A nucleic basic analysis can normally distinguish HIV the earliest (around 10 to 33 days after openness). Study the window time frame for every HIV test.

On the off chance that you think you've been presented to HIV as of now, converse with a medical services supplier, a trauma center specialist, or a pressing consideration supplier about post-openness prophylaxis (Energy) immediately.